THE FOETAL CIRCULATION

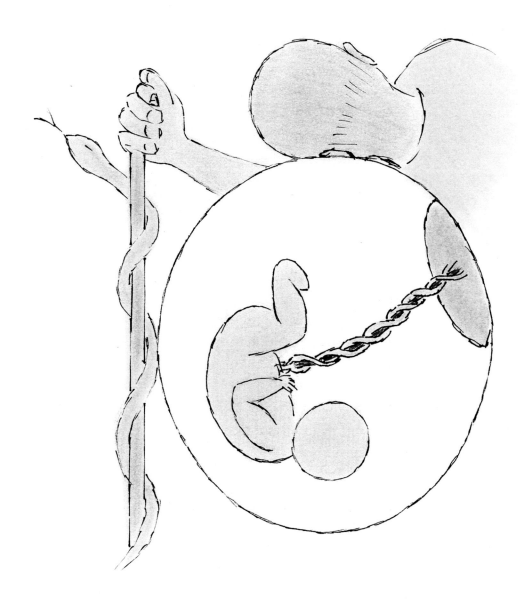

5th edition 2018

Alan Gilchrist

AuthorHouse™ UK
1663 Liberty Drive
Bloomington, IN 47403 USA
www.authorhouse.co.uk
Phone: 0800.197.4150

Published by AuthorHouse 08/29/2018

ISBN: 978-1-5462-9631-7 (sc)
ISBN: 978-1-5462-9632-4 (e)

Print information available on the last page.

Any people depicted in stock imagery provided by Getty Images are models, and such images are being used for illustrative purposes only. Certain stock imagery © Getty Images.

This book is printed on acid-free paper.

authorHOUSE®

THE FOETAL CIRCULATION

5th Edition 2018   *Alan Gilchrist*

Contents

This book is dedicated to the memory of my parents,
James and Ivy Gilchrist, and my wife Pauline.

Acknowledgements

I am grateful to my son Andrew for providing me with a room in his home, from where I have been able to compose my thoughts in comfort and peace, and to his wife Kim who has been a great help with my computer problems. They and their son Luke have helped me to transfer my mobile phone pictures on to my manuscript, and Ryan Price of E. E. Oswestry has done his best to help me too. I am especially grateful to Mrs Gill Darlington for helping me to find a sheep farmer near Oswestry, and to the farmer Graham Jones of Red House Farm for giving me four stillborn lambs. It is difficult to appreciate fully the value of their contribution to this publication. They have proved to be an important source of information on the human foetal circulation, and I do thank Graham Jones most sincerely for giving them so readily and for phoning me in the mornings when they had been delivered in the night. In parallel with the lamb dissections was the taking of pictures of them with my mobile phone cameras from Samsung and Nokia. I was surprised by the quality of the reproduction each one gave. I have acknowledged in the text part of an important article in the Journal of the British Institute of Radiology : 'A Radiographic Demonstration of the Circulation through the Heart in the Adult and in the Foetus, and the Identification of the Ductus Arteriosus'. I am grateful to the Institute for allowing me to publish it. Martyn Cooke, in charge of Conservation at the Royal College of Surgeons in London, had already given me permission to publish part of a letter concerning lung casts, in a previous version of my book. I thank him and his staff for taking the casts out of storage for me, and I regret I was unable to visit the College and see them. An article on ventricular wall thicknesses by Professor Calvin E. Oyer et al, is acknowledged in the text. I was very fortunate in being able to find a lady who would let me listen to her foetal heart. She has permitted me to include her name with the details of my Sunday morning visit to her. On 7th July 2018 Battams the butcher in Oswestry provided me with the heart lungs and liver of a lamb, all connected as I had asked. I am grateful for the valuable specimens that Battams has provided from time to time. John Quinn, photographer in Oswestry has reproduced all my diagrams drawings and photographs in high definition, and I do thank him for the quality of this special type of work.

References.

The Foetal Circulation. The Personal Account by a Zimbabwe Family Practitioner. By Alan Gilchrist. Printed in Zimbabwe by Graphtec Zimbabwe. 2011.

The Foetal Circulation Reflections. By Alan Gilchrist. Printed by YouCaxton Publications. 2015.

The Foetal Circulation. By Alan Gilchrist. Published by AuthorHouse. 2017.

Part 1. The Beginning and Information from the Animals.

I first heard about two different streams of blood; one arterial and the other venous, flowing in the right atrium of the heart without mixing, during a biology class when I was a medical student in London. I wondered how it was done. I must have carried the problem around with me, because more than 20 years later when I was working in Africa it was still bothering me. I was the medical superintendent of the hospital in Fort Victoria, the first white township established in Southern Rhodesia in 1890 by the Pioneers who had travelled up from South Africa. The town is now called Masvingo and the country is Zimbabwe. For three of the four years I worked there, I was single-handed. Then as well as doing the clinical work, I became involved with a huge amount of forensic medicine for the Police. In April 1965 a baby girl was delivered in the hospital under my care, and died because we were unable to make her breathe. Her body had been taken to the hospital mortuary, where not surprisingly I was performing a police post-mortem. I was engrossed with the autopsy, but my thoughts gradually turned towards her. If she had not breathed, would she be like a foetus in utero which does not breathe? Had we delivered a foetus, and would her organs still be in the foetal condition? So I finished the autopsy, went over to her and removed the heart and lungs together, put them in preserving fluid, took them home and later examined them. In the mortuary I noted the position of the heart which lay horizontally above the raised diaphragm, with the unexpanded lungs tucked back on either side. None of the accounts I have read mentions the raised diaphragm or the horizontal position of the heart. I assume it is the normal arrangement, contributing to the economy of space so important in the little curled up intrauterine creature. Diagram 1.

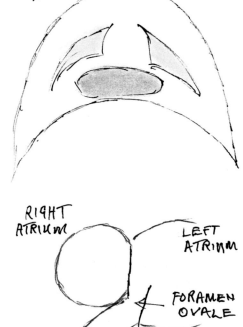

When I began to examine the specimen later at home, I could see how the streams were separated. It was a special moment for me; the first time I had examined a foetal heart which gave me the answers I was seeking. I had seen something never seen or described before. I thought I had been guided. The mouth of the upper end of the inferior vena cava, which was oval, was closely and accurately applied round the foramen ovale in the atrial septum, and therefore led into the left atrium, not the right. So in life the placental flow would have entered the left atrium directly without having entered the right atrium at all. The right atrium was in the shape of a tube lying above the inferior vena cava, and the venous return in that atrium would have flowed above the placental stream in the inferior vena cava below. I showed the specimen to my wife and explained how the streams were separated. She said 'It's like a flyover.' What an apt description. Diagram 2.

The ductus arteriosus did not lead into the aorta, as described in the orthodox accounts. Instead, both ductus and aorta were large vessels of the same size lying side by side with a narrow angle between them, and led into the descending aorta together. Diagram 3.

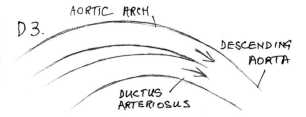

I realised that the orthodox accounts were wrong and had to be changed. That is why I decided to produce my own version. The first three diagrams here are copied from my first little book published in Zimbabwe in 2011.

My doubts about the accounts were strengthened on considering the separation of the two streams. The authors of the accounts probably knew; at least they should have known, that when two different levels of the respiratory gases meet, such as between the air and the lung capillaries, and between the peripheral tissues and their capillaries, rapid exchanges occur in a fraction of a second leading to equilibrium. The same reaction would occur in the meeting of arterial and venous blood in the same part of the heart, leading to a homogeneous mixture of them both. So in my book, and in subsequent versions, I considered that where there are different streams together, they would be separated in vessels containing either arterial or venous blood; not arterial and venous separated in the same vessel or chamber of the heart. This led me to believe that the blood in the pulmonary trunk would be pure venous and of no use to the foetal lungs. That is why I maintained that the lungs would be nourished only by the bronchial circulation. But I was wrong; there is a pulmonary circulation for the lungs, as I will show you from my examination of foetal lambs. It also led me to believe that there must be a block to prevent the venous return from the lower body from using the upper part of the inferior vena cava to reach the heart, otherwise it would have contaminated the placental stream leading to the left atrium. In this case I was partly correct; there must be a block to prevent the lower return from entering the left atrium, but there is some venous return from the liver which does join the placental stream. So without doubt a single stream of mixed blood in the upper inferior vena cava, mainly arterial from the placenta and partly venous from the liver, does enter the left atrium. I hope eventually to make all these things clearer.

Information from the Animals.

Since finding the foetal heart in the mortuary in 1965, I had believed that it is the foetus which is delivered, and that the baby is born after the delivery when the first deep breath is taken. So I was very interested in an animal programme on television which showed the birth of a foal, and I followed the events carefully. At first the non-breathing lifeless-looking form of the animal, with a narrow unexpanded chest was delivered on to the ground. Then almost immediately it took a deep breath and opened its chest, stood up on all four legs and shook itself. My belief was confirmed; I had seen a foetus changed into a foal.

In another animal programme on television, I watched the delivery of a goat kid. It emerged in a flaccid lifeless form and did not breathe. So it was stillborn, and I knew I had watched the delivery of a foetus. I realised then that stillborn farm animals could be a valuable source of information on the foetal circulation, if human foetuses were unavailable, and in February 2018 a sheep farmer near Oswestry kindly gave me four stillborn lambs during the lambing season. I examined each one as it became available and kept dissected parts in formalin. There was no room in my jars for the complete animals, so I had to amputate all the legs and remove the head before I could examine the viscera and later preserve them. I regretted this because I was unable to see the vascular system for the hind legs. The results of my examinations amazed me. I had completed the manuscript for the 5th edition of my book by January, but I had to change much of it and rewrite it after seeing the things revealed to me by the foetal lambs. I had included many diagrams in the original manuscript and I had to replace some of these too. At each stage I took pictures of my work with my mobile phone camera, and they have been inserted along with the diagrams to help you understand the text. The text and the diagrams may also help you to understand the pictures; they are all complementary. I did not take pictures in 1965; but I made accurate drawings of the inferior vena cava leading to the left atrium, which were lost in 1968 when I was examining human foetuses in our medical school. This was a big blow for me, which made it more difficult for my findings to be accepted by others. But now that I have been able to record photographically some crucially important findings in the foetal lambs, I am hopeful that they will be accepted as a true record. I had thought that all mammals would have a vascular system similar to our own. There are similarities, but there are differences too, as I will show you.

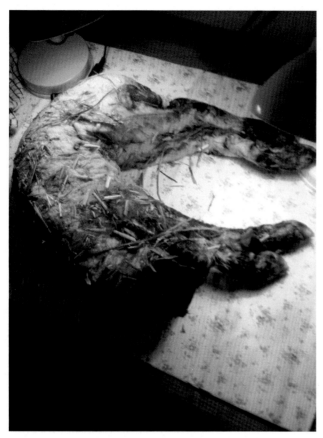

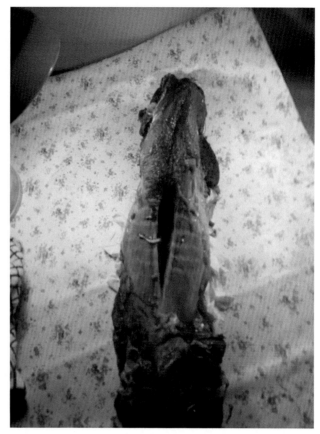

| Picture 1 | Picture 2 |

Picture 1 shows one of the stillborn foetal lambs and the straw of its delivery bed in the farm. I have specially included picture 2 to show you how narrow is a foetal lamb's chest before a deep breath is taken.

The first thing that surprised me was the liver; I learned a lot from the liver. There was no inferior vena cava below the liver, just a short vessel above it connected to the heart. The umbilical vein entered the liver near its middle and divided to reach all parts of the liver tissue. There was no part of the vein outside the liver such as a ductus venosus; only the one vessel entering the liver. The same liver tissue was drained by tributaries of the hepatic veins, which converged together between the upper surface of the liver and the under surface of the central tendon of the diaphragm. On the upper surface of the tendon the hepatic veins became the proximal end of the inferior vena cava, which led to the heart.

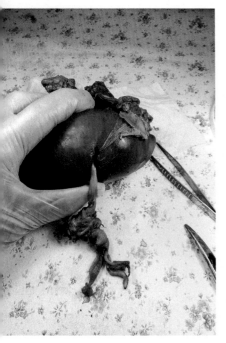
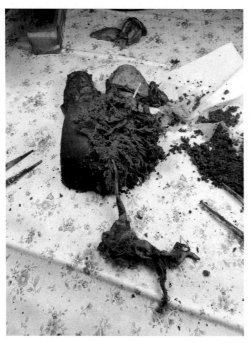
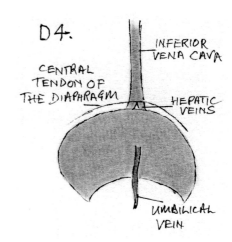
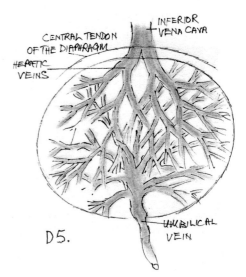

Picture 3   Picture 4

Picture 3 shows the umbilical vein entering the liver. Picture 4 shows the branches of the umbilical vein spreading out within the liver, and the stick in the inferior vena cava receiving the hepatic veins draining the liver tissues. Diagrams 4 and 5 may help to explain these things.

The inferior vena cava draining the liver was a much bigger vessel than the umbilical vein supplying it, and I realised the discrepancy was due to the additional blood supply for the liver from the hepatic artery and the blood in the portal vein draining the alimentary tract. I identified both vessels. Blood from both systems would eventually reach the hepatic veins and the inferior vena cava with the blood from the umbilical vein. *So the inferior vena cava would have carried a mixture of blood from three sources to the heart: the umbilical vein, the hepatic artery and the portal vein. But the components of the mixture would not have been separated; the mixture would have been homogeneous; any separation would have been separation of a part of the mixture and there would have been no streaming into arterial and venous, as commonly alleged in the orthodox accounts of the human.*

The foetal lamb and its liver tell us more about the circulation. The venous return from the upper body drains into the superior vena cava, which leads into the right atrium. The venous return from the lower body must also reach the right atrium, but it cannot use the inferior vena cava because there is no inferior vena cava below the liver to connect to. There must be an alternative route.

I had not intended to make a detailed study of the anatomy of a lamb; I was most interested in the foetal circulation. But as I proceeded with my examinations it became necessary to explore further. I thought there must be an azygos vein, but I could not find it. Before examining the heart and other internal viscera I had removed them from the vertebral column. Perhaps I had damaged the vein, I am not sure. In the various parts which I had removed from the four foetal lambs and preserved in formalin, there was no evidence of an azygos vein. All I could find was a collection of small veins beneath the pleura in the gutters on either side of the vertebral column. I really needed a fifth specimen to examine this question carefully, and the farmer phoned me to say there was one available. But on 18th March 2018 I had fallen badly in my room and damaged my back, and I was unable to fetch and work on this last valuable specimen. Then the lambing season finished. If I am able I will try to sort out this problem next year, but now I am in the process of completing my story and I must finish it without a few answers. However, on 28th June 2018 I rescued one of my old specimens containing the vertebral column, and explored it. There were several small veins in each paravertebral gutter. Also on each side was what appeared to be a large vessel. Each petered out below where they were fixed to a vertebra prominens. I opened them; they were not vessels, they were probably salivary glands. There was no clotted blood inside them, just some amorphous looking substance. I think the small veins in the paravertebral gutters would have been part of the venous drainage system for the lower body, but I am not sure if they should be called azygos veins.

Yes there must be an alternative indirect route, and perhaps those paravertebral veins are part of it. In the *postnatal human* the lower return has two routes to *the right* atrium: either directly via the inferior vena cava or indirectly via the azygos vein. But in the human *foetus* the direct route leads *into the left atrium* and must be closed to prevent the venous return from entering it, and the indirect route using the azygos vein, must be used. I must return to my original idea; that there must be a block in the inferior vena cava to prevent the lower return from contaminating the placental stream in the upper part. In the lamb the block is the absent vena cava below the liver; in the human the block is probably within the liver itself high up and squashed within the narrow chest. In both the foetal lamb and in the human foetus, therefore, the lower return would reach the right atrium indirectly through the superior vena cava, and in each case the superior vena cava would be reserved exclusively to carry the total venous return into the right atrium, while in each case the inferior vena cava above the liver would be reserved exclusively to carry the placental stream into the left atrium.

A.Z: AZYGOS VEIN
D.V: DUCTUS VENOSUS
F.O: FORAMEN OVALE
I.V.C: INFERIOR VENA CAVA
S.V.C: SUPERIOR VENA CAVA
U.V: UMBILICAL VEIN.

So, as I see it, in the human foetus the inferior vena cava is functionally separated by the liver into two parts. The lower part carries the lower return to the right atrium, and the upper part carries the placental stream to the left atrium; and though there would be some venous return joining the upper part from the liver itself, it should strictly not be called a vena cava, because it carries mainly *arterial* blood to the *left* atrium. Then the ductus venosus in the human foetus should strictly not be called a ductus if it does not carry the placental stream into a vena cava; it is really the upper part of the umbilical vein carrying the main stream of arterial blood to the left atrium. But it has to have a name, and it will be difficult to change the present well-establish one. Later on, during the birth changes, I will show you how the upper vessel will truly deserve to be called a vena cava. See diagram 6.

In the foetal lamb, (and also in the human foetus), It is unlikely for the liver to be the first organ supplied by the umbilical vein just because of its position. There is more to it than that. The umbilical vein does not pass through the liver in a single channel to the inferior vena cava; it divides and appears to meet the tributaries of the hepatic veins within the liver tissues. So what goes on in the liver; what happens to the oxygen? Some will be supplied by the hepatic artery; but that oxygen has already passed though the liver to the heart and beyond. *Whatever happens in the foetal lamb's liver, the oxygen which reaches the hepatic veins and inferior vena cava from the placenta must either have survived the passage through the liver, or been manufactured there.* You cannot deny that; there is no other supply of oxygen from a ductus venosus outside the liver to the lamb's inferior vena cava.

The upper part of the inferior vena cava leads to the side of the right atrium and ends in a small tunnel, at the bottom of which is the foramen ovale. For the second time in my life, 53 years after the first, I have seen the inferior vena cava leading directly to the foramen ovale and the left atrium. But this time I have been able to show it in a picture. Picture 5 shows the inferior vena cava, which I have opened, leading directly to the foramen ovale, and the superior vena cava above the heart leading to the right atrium, which I have also opened. The right ventricle is in front of the larger left ventricle. Diagram 7 helps to explain.

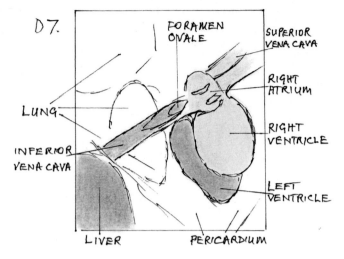

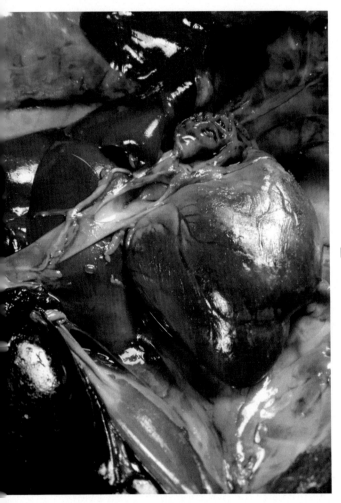

Picture 5

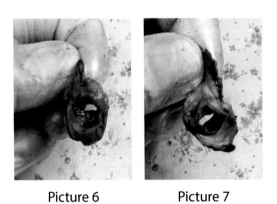

Picture 6   Picture 7

On each side of the foramen ovale is a recess surrounded by the thick muscle tissue of the interatrial wall. It was not easy to identify the septum secundum, though on the proximal side the floor of the tunnel was thickened into a 'V' shape, and beyond was a loose semi-circular membrane firmly attached at its edges to the wall of the tunnel, which I suppose was the septum primum. It had a strong sharp upper edge firmly anchored on each side. I removed the interatrial tissue above the valve and exposed the valve with the tunnel on one side and the recess in the left atrium on the other. In order to close the valve in atrial systole there would have to be two muscle actions; one to pull from side to side to stretch the membrane, and another to pull the upper edge of the membrane upwards to close the gap. The venous return in the right atrium from the superior vena cava would have passed over the blood flowing into the left atrium in a flyover manner. I removed the valve and took pictures from each side.

Picture 6 shows the valve from the left atrial side, while picture 7 shows it in the end of the tunnel.

6

Shortly before the end of the tunnel there is a gap in the inferior vena cava, which would allow some of the mainly arterial stream in the inferior vena cava to separate and enter the right atrium. I think there must be a valve guarding the gap, to prevent backflow in atrial systole. I could not be sure. On 7th June 2018, I explored the tunnel and neighbouring vessels of the foetal lambs' hearts.

In picture 8 the shorter stick is propping open the inferior vena cava, with the foramen ovale beyond in its recess at the end of the tunnel. The gap is beneath the short stick and leads into the right atrium, which I have opened. The longer stick is in the superior vena cava leading into the right atrium. I have pinned back the cut edge of the right atrium to expose the gap, with the entrance to a smaller tunnel beneath it.

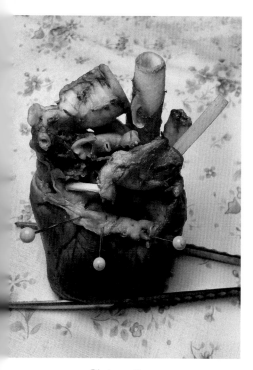
Picture 8

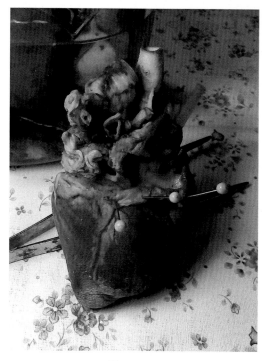
Picture 9

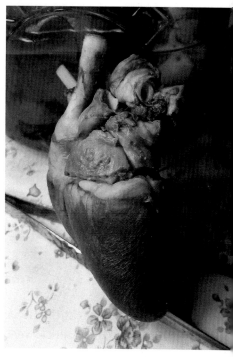
Picture 10

I opened the smaller tunnel, picture 9, and followed it as it narrowed and led into the groove between the left atrium and ventricle, Picture 10. There were tiny dots in its wall which meant small blood vessels leading off it. Then the penny dropped; it was the coronary sinus draining the venous return from the heart itself into the right atrium. In atrial diastole the openings of the coronary sinus, the inferior vena cava and superior vena cava would allow blood to enter the right atrium, while the foramen ovale would admit blood into the left atrium. In systole the inflows would stop as blood would be ejected into the ventricles. Without doubt the centre for control of the circulation in the foetal lamb was nearby.

From the right atrium the venous blood, now carrying some of the mainly arterial blood from the inferior vena cava, would enter the right ventricle and be pumped into the pulmonary trunk. This is a large vessel issuing from the right ventricle, larger than the aorta issuing by its side from the left ventricle. A single vessel arose from the aorta; the only one supplying the upper body. I have called it cephalic for want of a better name. It divided into several smaller branches. From the underside of the pulmonary trunk there was a bulge from which the pulmonary arteries arose on each side. The shorter one entered the left lung, while the longer right artery passed between the aorta in front and the trachea behind to enter the right lung; dividing into one main artery and two smaller branches before entry. Beyond the origins of the cephalic and pulmonary arteries, the aorta and the terminal part of the pulmonary trunk known as the ductus arteriosus, lay close to each other side by side and merged together at a junction to form the beginning of the descending aorta, as I had seen in the human in 1965. In this case the aorta was larger than the ductus. Picture 11, and diagram 8, show the left pulmonary artery leading off the pulmonary trunk and the cephalic artery arising from the aorta. The ductus arteriosus and aorta then join to form the descending aorta.

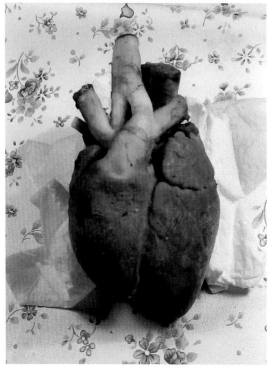

Picture 11

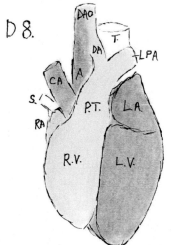

A: AORTA. CA: CEPHALIC ARTERY
DA: DUCTUS ARTERIOSUS. DAO: DESCENDING
AORTA. LA: LEFT ATRIUM. LPA: LEFT
PULMONARY ARTERY. LV: LEFT
VENTRICLE. P.T: PULMONARY TRUNK
RA: RIGHT ATRIUM. RV: RIGHT
VENTRICLE. S: STICK IN SUPERIOR
VENA CAVA. T: TRACHEA.

The blood from the pulmonary arteries feeding the lungs would return in the pulmonary veins to the left atrium, and re-join the arterial stream there which had passed through the foramen ovale. In one of the lambs I could see the two left pulmonary veins, full of blood at their entrance to the left atrium. *So there would have been a pulmonary circulation for the lungs.*

I opened the aorta, the pulmonary trunk and their branches up to the descending aorta, and measured their internal circumferences with my mini Vernier calliper. These are the results, shown alongside diagram 9.

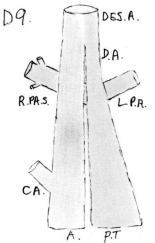

A. AORTA C. CEPHALIC ARTERY
D.A. DUCTUS ARTERIOSUS
DES.A. DESCENDING AORTA
L.PA. LEFT PULMONARY ARTERY
P.T. PULMONARY TRUNK
R.PAS. RIGHT PULMONARY ARTERIES.

Aorta at its origin: 21.65mm.

Pulmonary trunk at its origin: 24.6mm.

Cephalic artery: 9.1mm.

Left pulmonary artery: 9.6mm.

Right main pulmonary artery: 10.2mm.

Smaller right pulmonary artery: 4.6mm.

Smallest right pulmonary artery: 3.75mm.

Ductus just before the junction: 8.4mm.

Aorta just before the junction: 14.35mm.

Descending aorta just after the junction: 17.5mm.

I was surprised by the large size of the pulmonary arteries compared with the cephalic artery. Even the smaller of the two vessels for the lungs, the left pulmonary artery, is larger than the vessel supplying the head, brain and upper limb. However, the level of oxygen and food in the blood passing through the lungs would be very low, and the rate of flow required would be very high. Also, at birth the two vessels will have to share all the blood in the circulation passing from the pulmonary trunk to the expanded lungs. The aorta before the junction is larger than the ductus, which would seem to indicate a good supply of arterial blood for the lower body and placenta. But with the large supply to the lungs there would be an equivalent return of venous blood to the left atrium, reducing the oxygen concentration there.

From diagram 9, I have developed another, showing the sections of the foetal circulation with the two crossover transfers of blood from one side to the other: mainly arterial from the inferior vena cava to the right atrium, mainly venous from the pulmonary trunk to the lungs and venous from the lungs to the left atrium. The blue foetus indicates its venous return. After the crossovers the streams would be mainly arterial and mainly venous, and the descending aorta a blend of the two. Diagram 10.

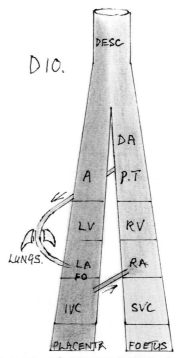

Another surprise for me was the larger size of the pulmonary trunk compared with the aorta. Since seeing the rolled up position of the right atrium in 1965 I had always considered the right atrium (and ventricle) to be smaller than the left atrium (and ventricle). But now, because of the vessel measurements, I may have to change my ideas; is it the other way round? We must not forget what we learned in the anatomy room, that the right atrioventricular opening admits three fingers and the tricuspid valve has three cusps, while the left atrioventricular opening admits two fingers and the mitral valve has only two cusps. However, there may be other things to consider such as the speed of the flows in the aorta and pulmonary trunk. Would they be the same? Or would the aortic flow be faster, ensuring an adequate supply for the upper body structures, in spite of the small size of the cephalic artery?

A. AORTA DA. DUCTUS ARTERIOSUS
DESC. DESCENDING AORTA
FO. FORAMEN OVALE IVC. INFERIOR VENA CAVA
LA. LEFT ATRIUM LV. LEFT VENTRICLE
PT. PULMONARY TRUNK RA. RIGHT ATRIUM
RV. RIGHT VENTRICLE SVC. SUPERIOR VENA CAVA

We all know, or should know, that in the postnatal state the pulmonary arteries carry only *venous* blood from the body tissues to the peripheral respiratory zone, where the respiratory exchanges occur, and *oxygenated* blood returns to the left atrium in the pulmonary veins. In the foetus the remarkable opposite occurs; the pulmonary arteries are utilised to carry a mixture of venous and *arterial* blood to the lungs, and the pulmonary veins return *venous* blood to the left atrium, contaminating the placental stream there. The nutrition of the foetal lungs would therefore be supplied by both pulmonary and bronchial circulations, but in the postnate the supply would come from the bronchial only, because blood returning from the respiratory zone in the pulmonary veins would contain only oxygen, no food.

So what have we learned from the foetal lambs?

1 In the lamb there is no inferior vena cava below the liver.

2 In the foetal lamb the inferior vena cava above the liver carries the placental stream into the left atrium, as I have seen in the human foetus.

3 In the foetal lamb the venous return from the lower body must reach the right atrium by another indirect route, possibly by paravertebral veins and the superior vena cava.

4 In the human foetus the lower venous return uses the azygos vein as the indirect route to the superior vena cava and the right atrium.

5 In the human foetus the liver separates the inferior vena cava functionally into two parts; the upper part to carry the placental stream to the left atrium and the lower part to carry the lower return to the right atrium.

6 The placental stream carries a mixture of mainly arterial, and venous, blood.

7 In the foetal lamb a part of the placental stream passes through a gap in the inferior vena cava into the right atrium.

8 In both species the inferior vena cava above the liver is not a vena cava; it is a vessel reserved exclusively to carry the mainly arterial placental stream into the left atrium.

9 In both species the superior vena cava is a vessel reserved exclusively to carry the total venous return from the foetus into the right atrium.

10 The foetal lamb does not have a ductus venosus.

11 The ductus venosus in the human foetus is not a ductus; it is part of the umbilical vein.

12 In both species the ductus arteriosus is not a ductus. It lies side by side with the aorta and both vessels enter the descending aorta together.

13 In the foetal lamb the ductus is much smaller than the aorta

14 In the foetal lamb there is a generous pulmonary circulation for the foetal lungs, which supplies nutrition as well as oxygen.

15 After birth the postnatal human has an alternative direct route for the lower return to reach the right atrium via the inferior vena cava, but the lamb has only the indirect foetal route.

16 In both species each atrium has its own separate blood supply: venous blood for the right atrium and arterial for the left.

17 In both species the venous return in the right atrium 'flies over' the arterial blood entering the left atrium.

18 In the foetal lamb the pulmonary trunk is larger than the aorta.

****

The fundamental error in the orthodox accounts is a large one with three components: separated streaming of arterial and venous blood, entering the right atrium, and the arterial stream passing through the foramen ovale from the right to left atrium. I recognised it in April 1965 when I examined a human foetal heart. I was correct when I refused to accept that the two streams could remain separate; my fundamental error was denying that there could be two streams entering the same chamber of the heart. It was a new concept for me. This was revealed to me in February 2018 when I was examining foetal lambs' hearts and saw the inferior vena cava carrying the placental stream to the left atrium. It had come from the liver and must have contained the venous return from the liver. Having been able to separate fact from fiction in each account; mine and theirs, I have been encouraged to produce a fresh version which I hope will be nearer the truth.

Part 2. The Human Foetal Circulation.

We can now begin our travels round the human foetal circulation. It is all about the way the placenta replaces the non-functional foetal lungs; supplies the foetus with oxygen and food and removes carbon dioxide and waste. But we must not forget the contribution from the mother during the gestation period (and beyond). It has been her blood, food and oxygen which have been transmitted to the placenta. She eats and breathes for the foetus and purifies its blood. Her own source of fresh air is the trees, which have a peripheral leafy green respiratory zone similar to her own, except that it not only respires continuously, but during the daylight hours absorbs carbon dioxide from the air and replaces it with oxygen. So there is one respiratory cycle between the trees and the mother, and another between the mother and the foetus. Diagram 11.

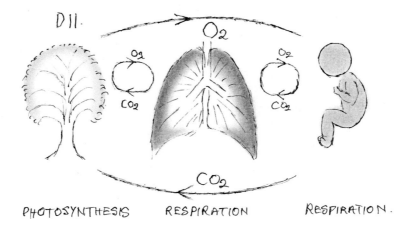

PHOTOSYNTHESIS   RESPIRATION   RESPIRATION.

Diagram 12 shows all the principal features of the foetal circulation numbered.

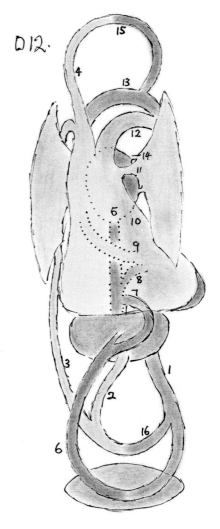

The right side of the heart is prominently shown with small parts of the left atrium behind the pulmonary trunk, and the tip of the left ventricle at the cardiac apex. The descending aorta (1) supplies the placenta and the lower body with mixed arterial and venous blood (16). The lower inferior vena cava (2) draining the lower body, connects with the azygos vein (3) which carries the lower return to the superior vena cava, (4) then continues to the liver where it is blocked. The upper inferior vena cava drains the liver and leads to the foramen ovale at the edge of the left atrium (5). The umbilical vein (6) carrying arterial blood from the placenta also leads to the liver where a small branch joins the portal vein, but the main vessel passes outside the liver and ends as the ductus venosus (7) in the inferior vena cava above the liver. A stream from the inferior vena cava (8) carries the arterial blood into the right atrium where it mixes with the venous flow from the superior vena cava (9), while most of the blood from the placenta continues in the upper inferior vena cava to the left atrium (5). The mixed mainly venous blood in the right atrium enters the right ventricle and is pumped up the pulmonary trunk (10). Some passes through the pulmonary arteries (11) to the lungs, while the remainder flows through the ductus arteriosus (12) side by side with the aorta (13) into the descending aorta. Venous blood returning from the lungs ends in the left atrium (14). The upper body (15) is supplied with mainly arterial blood, while the lower body (16) and placenta receive mixed.

Number 8, the stream from the inferior vena cava deserves an explanation. In the lambs I had found a gap in the vena cava which permitted the right atrium to receive arterial blood destined for the lungs. But I know of no such connection between the inferior vena cava and the right atrium in the human. However, in the previous version of my book I said 'I don't think the vena cava is fused with the septum; otherwise, it would have to be torn away at birth and would be an impediment. It would appear to be held against the septum, probably by muscular action of the right atrium, especially in systole. If there was a leak at the junction, it would not matter if it was small. It would only result in the addition of some arterial blood from the inferior vena cava entering the right atrium,' etc. So now I believe that a leak in atrial diastole is the actual method in the human for adding arterial blood to the venous for the benefit of the lungs. Diagram 13. In support of this belief is an article in the British Journal of Radiology 1939 12: 141, 505-517 by A. E. Barclay, Sir Joseph Barcroft, D. H. Barron, and K. J. Franklin, which states 'a minor part of the inferior caval blood passes with the superior caval flow into the right (atrium and) ventricle and out into the pulmonary arteries and, via the ductus arteriosus, into the descending aorta.' They had demonstrated it radiographically. (My brackets; the blood must first pass through the atrium before reaching the ventricle).

I have shown by examining the hearts of a human foetus and foetal lambs, that the blood supply for the heart travelling in the upper inferior vena cava, enters the left atrium not the right. This not only contradicts the standard accounts, which say that the inferior vena cava enters the right atrium, but shows that each atrium has its own separate supply: venous blood for the right atrium and arterial blood for the left, as in the baby. The hole in the atrial septum may have suggested lateral flow, but the flow is from the inferior vena

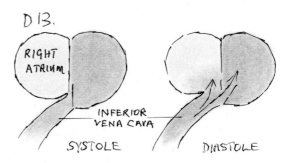

cava, not from the right atrium. *Whether it be from the lungs of the baby or the placenta of the foetus, the oxygen from the respiratory organ goes direct to the left heart. It is a principle.*

I have also shown in human and lambs' foetal hearts how the venous return in the right atrium from the superior vena cava flows above the placental stream entering the left atrium. This is the flyover; it is one of the two foundation stones of my plan of the foetal circulation. Diagrams 14 and 15.

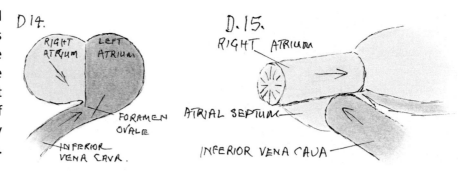

The foramen ovale guarding the entrance to the left atrium, is the first part of the heart reached by the placental stream in the inferior vena cava. It consists of two septa: primum and secundum, fused together below and separated above, movement between them allowing blood to pass into the left atrium. The oval hole is the cut out part of septum secundum on the right side, covered on the left by septum primum, as shown in diagram 16.

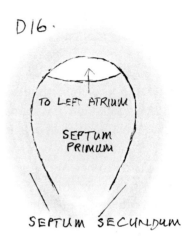

I have three drawings of the valve which I made in 1968 when I was examining foetuses in our medical school. 'A' shows the valve in the medial wall of the right atrium. 'B' shows the interior of the left atrium, with the atrioventricular opening on the left and the foramen ovale on the right. 'C' gives a good view of septum primum in the medial wall of the left atrium, with the upper part of secundum beyond.

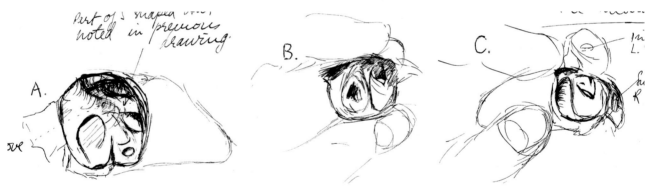

It would appear from the drawings that the septa are part of the muscular atrial septum, and that in atrial systole contraction of the septa would close the gap between the two and eject blood into the left ventricle. In an earlier version of my book I had suggested a principle where inlet valves open actively and outlet valves open passively by the pressure of the blood flow. In which case it would seem that the foramen ovale, being an inlet valve, would both open and close actively by muscular action of the septal wall. It is not a little flap valve buffeted hither and thither by the blood stream, as described in some of the orthodox accounts, which would make it an impediment to the low pressure stream. It is an active valve opening and closing actively, and is more likely to cause movement of blood rather than be moved by it.

I have several ideas about the foramen ovale, and will reveal some of them. The two atria lie close together, being parts of the biventricular heart. The right heart benefits from the coronary circulation from the left ventricle, and the left heart shares the cardiac impulse from the pacemaker in the right atrium. If we consider the two foetal atria and the two atria of the postnatal heart, the only one of the four atria to have an inlet valve is the foetal left atrium. The function of the inlet valve is to allow a measured amount of blood into the left atrium in atrial diastole, and prevent backflow in atrial systole. So the other three must prevent backflow in a different way. There may be various ways in which this is accomplished by the three, but there is a factor common to all four, which is the powerful suction by the ventricles during ventricular diastole which helps the atria to pump blood forwards in their systole. The postnatal left atrium is also helped by the force of the right ventricle pumping blood through the lungs to the atrium at a rate five times faster than the respiratory rate. The foetal left atrium does not have this help because the lungs are out of action and the blood supply comes from another direction, from the two ventricles pumping together in parallel, but the journey to the placenta and back is a long and precarious one. By the time the blood in the umbilical vein has reached the left atrium its pressure would be very low; probably the lowest in the circulation, and without a valve at the entrance to the atrium the blood supply to the heart would be haphazard. The pacemaker guarantees a steady flow of blood from the heart, but it is the foramen ovale, guided by the pacemaker, which ensures a constant flow of blood to the heart itself. *That is the reason for the valve; to ensure a constant supply of blood for the heart. It has absolutely nothing to do with 'shunting' blood from one side of the heart to the other.* At birth the two septa will be closed, separating the atria, and providing the blood a smooth passage through them without any impediments to the flows.

The authors of the orthodox accounts have a problem trying to explain how the arterial part of the mixed blood in the right atrium passes into the left atrium. I suppose they know that for a flow to occur between two heart chambers, each must beat in sequence; first the one then the other, such as between the atria and ventricles. But the atria do not beat in sequence, they beat at the same time together, and there cannot be a flow from one to the other. Also, the direction of the valve indicates that the pressure in the left atrium would be higher than in the right atrium, and the function of the valve would be to prevent backflow from the left to right atrium. The authors get over this dilemma by assuming the pressure in the right atrium to be higher than that in the left atrium and say that the blood 'is shunted through, enters through, is directed through, passes through, flows through,' without mentioning the words 'pumped through,' and ignoring the direction of the valve. This would mean that the 'little flap valve' would be held open throughout the gestation period, making not a sound until it is closed at birth. But there is a sound as the valve closes with each beat of the heart, as any lady in the later months of pregnancy may confirm with a Doppler foetal heart monitor.

The two sounds made by the postnatal heart measure the duration of ventricular systole, with the softer 'lub' heard as the ventricles contract and close the atrioventricular valves, and the harsher 'dup' occurring when the ventricles begin to open and the outlet valves close. The left ventricular sounds are louder than the right sounds, and we need only to consider them. The atrioventricular valve is the mitral and the outlet is the aortic.

In the foetus there is an extra sound made by the closing of the foramen ovale. It is much softer than the other two and more difficult to hear, because atrial muscle is much weaker than ventricular muscle, and when the left atrium contracts in systole the closing valve causes little vibration in the valve and the surrounding blood. But it can be heard nevertheless, and it occurs just before the other two as the atrium contracts immediately before the onset of ventricular systole. So there will be a triple rhythm; soft lub, louder lub, and harsher dup. Anybody with a Doppler machine should be able to find this rhythm, and it is best not to search for the individual sounds close together at a speed of 140 beats per minute; just find the triple gallop rhythm. Move the machine about and you will find the difference between the double

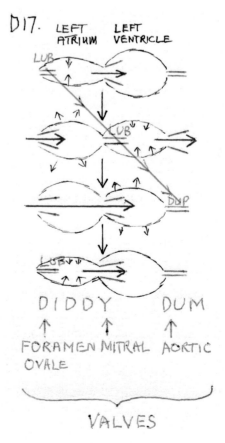

rhythm heard in some places and the gallop rhythm heard elsewhere: diddy-dum, diddy-dum, diddy-dum, with a very short diddy. See my diagram 17, of the foetal heart sounds.

On 19th November 2017 I was able to listen with my Doppler to the foetal heart in Nicola Pilgrim in Oswestry. I easily heard the triple gallop rhythm, even without my hearing aid as Nicola pointed out to me, and she and her husband heard it too. On the right side of the abdomen I could only hear the double rhythm, but on the left I picked up the gallop quickly. I did not examine Nicola otherwise, and did not give her any medical advice; I only explained why there should be the triple rhythm I was searching for. So my visit on that Sunday morning to a lady who was not a patient of mine, and in the cause of medical science, was not unethical. I was so grateful to her, and so excited. I bubbled over in the taxi going home.

It was so important to find the triple rhythm; it reveals so much. *It shows that the foetal heart has an extra valve, and that it is specifically the left atrium which is beating throughout pregnancy.* The right atrium is beating too of course, but it does not have an inlet valve to contribute to the heart sounds. So there must be a flow into the left atrium with each beat, *but not from the right atrium,* as I have said already, and it can only come from the placental stream in the inferior vena cava.

I think I may have begun to be interested in valves because of my own atrial fibrillation. In a healthy heart the mitral is a mixed valve; outlet for the left atrium and inlet for the left ventricle, and it would be pushed open weakly by the atrial blood pressure and pulled open by the chordae tendineae of the strong ventricular muscles. But with atrial fibrillation the ventricle would get no assistance from the malfunctioning atrium in ventricular diastole, and the left ventricle would be working alone to open the valve and suck the blood forward. So it would have to do work in both systole and diastole, and we have to abandon the concept of heart muscle working in systole and relaxing in diastole. There must be two sets of cardiac muscle, one contracting and the other relaxing at the same time. In systole one set would contract and close the ventricle while the other relaxes, then in diastole the second set would contract and open the ventricle while the first relaxes. (Perhaps we may have to reconsider the interpretation of the electrocardiogram; could the biphasic RS component be due to the double muscular action I have just described?)

Having passed through the foramen ovale into the left atrium, the mainly arterial stream enters the left ventricle and is pumped into the aorta, where five large vessels are given off: the coronary arteries, the brachiocephalic trunk, the left common carotid artery and the left subclavian artery. The venous blood in the right ventricle, joined by the arterial portion from the upper inferior vena cava, is pumped up the pulmonary trunk where the two pulmonary arteries arise together from its underside. The trunk then continues side by side with the aorta and merges with it to form the beginning of the descending aorta. Though the distal part of the pulmonary trunk carries mainly venous blood, it has been named the 'ductus arteriosus' because it has the structure of an artery, and it has this structure because the pressure inside it is high, perhaps almost as high as the pressure in the aorta. So the word 'arteriosus' is appropriate, but not 'ductus' as I have shown in part one, and will explain again later. The junction of the aorta with the 'ductus' is the other foundation stone of my plan.

These two unique foetal features; the flyover and the junction lay open before us the foundation of the plan of the foetal circulation. All we need do to see the whole plan is to add the upper, lower and placental sections. Diagram 18.

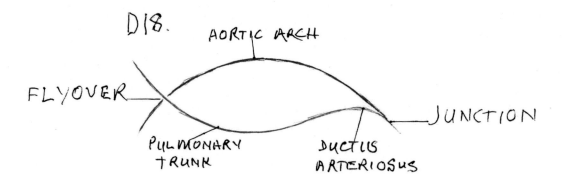

D18.

AORTIC ARCH

FLYOVER

JUNCTION

PULMONARY
TRUNK

DUCTUS
ARTERIOSUS

The junction has been misunderstood, and could not have been seen by those who have described it. It is often shown with the 'ductus' entering the aorta at almost a right angle, and sometimes the 'ductus' is smaller than the aorta. Diagram 19.

What I saw in 1965 was quite different, as I have already said. Both vessels were large, of the same size and lay side by side with a small angle between them. They converged together and merged into a single vessel that was the descending aorta. So we must be quite clear on this point; neither vessel enters the other; they lie side by side almost like the twin barrels of a double-barrelled shot gun and enter the aorta together, to form a single stream containing a mixture of arterial and venous blood. Diagram 20.

The two vessels are derivatives of the primitive aortic arches; the aorta from the 4th arch and the pulmonary trunk from the 6th. (The 5th arch is said to disappear completely, but I suspect that it may have developed into the two coronary arteries). Diagram 21.

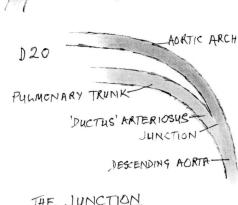

D19.

'DUCTUS' ARTERIOSUS

D20

AORTIC ARCH

PULMONARY TRUNK

'DUCTUS' ARTERIOSUS

JUNCTION

DESCENDING AORTA

THE JUNCTION

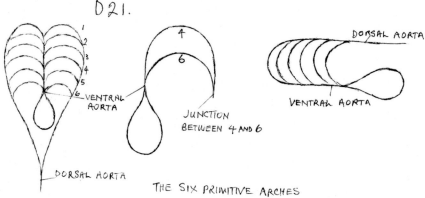

D21.

VENTRAL AORTA

DORSAL AORTA

JUNCTION
BETWEEN 4 AND 6

DORSAL AORTA

VENTRAL AORTA

THE SIX PRIMITIVE ARCHES

I suppose the concept of a ductus arose because of the mistaken way it was thought to enter the aorta, and it was only natural to think of the stream as a shunt. In support of these two misconceptions is the anatomy of the junction after birth when the ductus is now called the ligamentum arteriosum. I have dissected that part of a lamb's anatomy. The ligamentum does look like a ductus and suggests there would have been a shunt, but in the foetal lamb before birth there is neither ductus nor shunt. Diagram 22 shows my sketch of a lamb's ligamentum arteriosum.

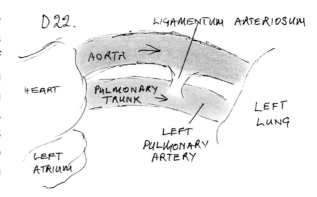

The concept of a ductus arteriosus leading into the foetal aorta is a complete myth; the primitive arches were never connected like this. However there is some advantage in retaining the name (it has to have one), providing that those who do so understand how it lies at the side of the aorta and does not enter it.

In 1968 I was allowed to dissect foetuses in the anatomy department of our medical school, and I made several drawings there. In drawing 'D' I have removed the heart and shown the structures which pass through the parietal pericardium. It is worth spending some time to study its interesting features. Note how the aorta (A) and the ductus arteriosus (DA), of the same size lie side by side. Also note the prominent pulmonary arteries arising together from the underside of the pulmonary trunk at the proximal end of the ductus. The roughly drawn line round the entrances of the pulmonary veins indicates where the attachment of the left atrium would have been. Notice the somewhat flattened outlines of the venae cavae compared

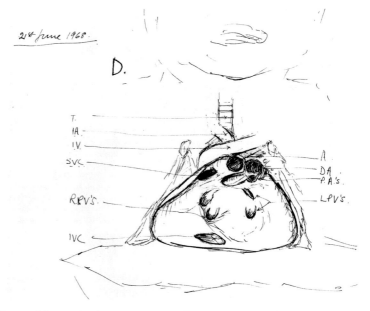

with the circular outlines of the arteries. (I.A. and I.V., old terminology; no names).

We have now demolished the false concepts of ductus venosus, ductus arteriosus and the shunting of blood from one side of the heart to the other. Perhaps they should all be laid to rest forevermore.

I had often driven through a road junction in Harare where two lanes of traffic converged into one, and the speed of the vehicles in the single lane ahead was twice (or more) the speed of the double stream behind. Diagram 23. This reminded me of the junction in the foetus where two streams joined into one, and I assumed the speed of the blood flowing down the descending aorta after the junction, would be twice as fast as the speed in each of the streams meeting at the junction. I then remembered that Dr David Clain had told me about the Venturi Principle or Effect, which concerns the increased speed and lowered pressure in a stream of liquid flowing through a narrow section of a tube. (Giovanni Venturi 1797).

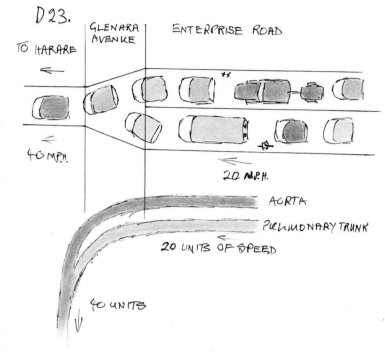

The junction would therefore segregate the blood supply of the upper body coming off the aorta before the junction, from the supply for the lower body and placenta flowing down the descending aorta. That for the upper body would be at high pressure, with a full complement of oxygen and food, low in carbon dioxide and waste (if any), and flowing at a certain speed. The mixed stream beyond the junction would be at lower pressure, with less oxygen and food, an increased amount of carbon dioxide and waste, and flowing at twice the speed of the other.

The upper circulation.

Diagram 24 shows the most important part of the circulation between the two unique foetal features; the flyover and the junction, which permits many privileged structures on the upper route to be supplied with oxygenated blood from the proximal aorta, and which emphasises the importance of them in the assembly of the new creature. The venous return enters the superior vena cava and right atrium.

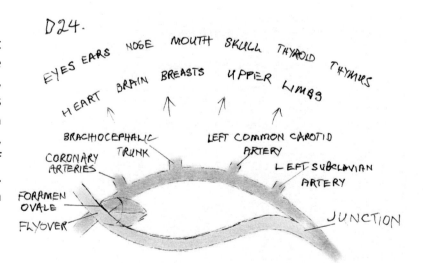

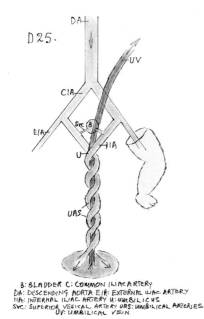

B: BLADDER C: COMMON ILIAC ARTERY
DA: DESCENDING AORTA E/A: EXTERNAL ILIAC ARTERY
IIA: INTERNAL ILIAC ARTERY U: UMBILICUS
SVC: SUPERIOR VESICAL ARTERY UAS: UMBILICAL ARTERIES
UV: UMBILICAL VEIN

The circulation for the lower body.

The mixed stream flowing down the descending aorta supplies the lower body and placenta.The stream for the lower body supplies the body wall, abdominal and pelvic viscera and the lower limbs. Diagram 25.

The venous return from the body wall travels in the hemiazygos system to the azygos vein, superior vena cava and right atrium, while the return from the viscera and lower limbs flows in the lower inferior vena cava to the azygos vein, superior vena cava and right atrium, and the total return from the foetus would enter the right atrium; leaving the left atrium free to be occupied by the mainly arterial placental stream. Diagram 26

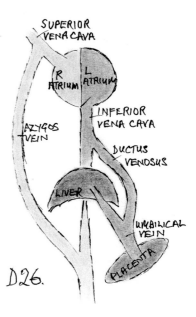

The Postnatal Lung.

Before discussing the circulation for the placenta, I want to introduce the postnatal lung and compare its features with those of the placenta.

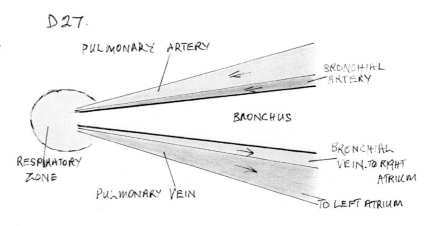

The lung has a dual blood supply: bronchial to supply its structure and pulmonary to meet its function of transporting the respiratory gases. The bronchial vessels bring arterial blood and depart with venous, while the pulmonary bring venous and depart with arterial. The bronchial veins drain into the azygos system and right atrium, and the pulmonary veins drain directly into the left atrium. The main bronchi at the root of the lung divide continually towards the lung periphery until the terminal bronchioles are reached leading into the respiratory tissues. The large pulmonary arteries at the root of the lung bringing in pure venous blood, can have no oxygen for themselves or the bronchi and surrounding lung tissue. It must be supplied by the bronchial arteries which run alongside the bronchi up to the terminal bronchioles. Beyond these the respiratory tissues of the respiratory zone receive oxygen from the air. Perhaps the smallest pulmonary veins leaving the periphery of the lung and their surrounding connective tissues will benefit from the oxygen they carry, and even the lining of the veins will benefit too. But if the connective tissues of the lungs further away from the pulmonary veins cannot benefit from the oxygen in those vessels, they must rely on oxygen brought by the bronchial vessels. That is how I see the relation between the two lung circulations; bronchial for the bronchi and connective tissues of the lungs, and pulmonary for the tissues of the body, (with perhaps a little for the lungs as well). Diagram 27.

In 1953 I visited the John Hunter Museum in the Royal College of Surgeons in London, and saw two beautiful casts of the lungs there. The bronchi and pulmonary vessels had been injected with resin and the other tissues had been removed with acid. I noticed a pattern in the relationships between the bronchi and the vessles, but there was no description of it nearby. In 2012 when I was living in Zimbabwe I wrote to the Curator of the Museum, and asked if the casts were still there. In part of his reply he said 'We do indeed have numerous examples of resin casts of the lung that were prepared by Dr David Tompsett. Dr Tompsett continued to prepare his amazing casts until he retired in the early 1980's.' I have not seen another description of the pattern I noticed, so I am now describing what I saw in 1953.

If you take a key ring and hold it horizontally, then you can pull out a key on each side. Imagine the keys to be the bronchi painted green, with the pulmonary arteries in blue lying above them, and the pulmonary veins in red lying below. Now without twisting the keys you can find the relationship of the bronchi and vessels in any part of the lungs. For example with the right lung, swing the right key up vertically. The pulmonary artery will lie medial to the bronchus and the vein laterally. Swing it down vertically through 180 degrees; the artery will be lateral and the vein medial. Swing it round to the front of the ring; the artery will lie in front of the bronchus with the vein behind. Swing it up through 180 degrees; the artery will lie behind with the vein in front. Swing it round to the back of the ring; the artery will be in front with the vein behind. Swing it down through 180 degrees; the artery will be behind with the vein in front. These manoeuvres can be repeated on the left side to give a mirror image of the positions in the right lung. The exercise could be repeated using a small fan, with the unexpanded blades held horizontally, with blue paint on the top and red paint below on each blade. Open the fan into a semi-circle and swivel it forwards and backwards with the same result as with the keys. I noticed that the arteries followed this pattern fairly faithfully, but the relationship of the veins to the bronchi was not so constant. In the upper lobes the bronchi and vessels were crowded together, but in the lower lobes there was more space between them. In the upper lobes the arteries would lie central to the bronchi, with the veins lying peripherally. In the lower lobes the arteries would lie on the outside of the bronchi and the veins on the inner side, with a gradual change from above downwards. Diagram 28.

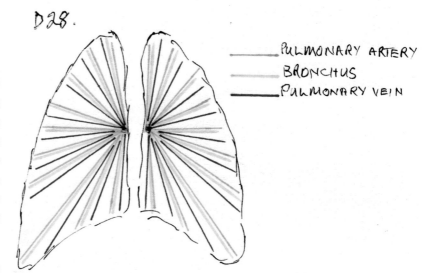

D28.

PULMONARY ARTERY
BRONCHUS
PULMONARY VEIN

Several years ago when I was living in Zimbabwe I tried to confirm what I had seen in 1953, by dissecting lungs which had been kept in preserving fluid, but when I removed the tissues between the bronchi and vessels there was no support to keep them in place, and they just became a loose tangled mess, which looked like a fly-whisk.

I had recently contacted the Royal College again and asked for permission to see the casts, but the Museum was being renovated and the specimens had been placed in storage for three years. However I have since been allowed to see them and they are being taken out of storage. Then I had a fall which has injured my back and I am more or less housebound and unable to visit the College.

I had hoped that by confirming the anatomy of the adult lung, I could assume a similar contracted version would be present in the foetal lung. But now I will make some slices through the foetal to see if they will confirm the arrangement in the adult lung.

On 24th May 2018 I examined the right lung of one foetal lamb. But I did not make accurate descriptions of the positions of the various sections, and even my pictures taken with my phone camera did not help. The next day I was more careful when I examined the left lung. I did not make cuts; I just removed the pleura and lung tissue from the inner vertebral surface of the lung from above downwards, and uncovered the bronchi and vessels. In the upper part only the arteries were visible; they covered the bronchi which lay lateral to them. Further down in the middle section the bronchi came into view below the arteries. In the lowest part the veins were prominent and obstructed the view of the bronchi. Diagram 29.

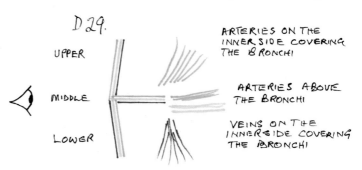

What I have seen so far in the lung of the foetal lamb, confirms what I saw in the museum in 1953. So it would appear that David Tompsett's work with lung casts has given us important information about the anatomy of the lung, which should be recognised as such by the medical profession. I would suggest that those of us who are interested in lung anatomy should visit the Royal College when the renovations have been completed, and study the lung casts.

The placenta and its circulation.

I liken the placenta to a dialysis machine which purifies the foetal blood. It is in two parts: maternal and foetal. The smaller maternal part embedded in the wall of the uterus provides the purified blood from the mother which is given to the foetus, while the larger foetal part receives the purified blood and gives venous to the maternal side in return. The foetal side is supplied with two streams of blood from the foetus, one venous from the right heart and the other arterial from the left heart. So in this respect it resembles the lung with streams of arterial and venous blood. The venous is for purification, as in the lung, and the arterial is most probably for the placenta itself. The placenta is a working organ and requires food and oxygen like any other working part. But the blood does not come in separated form, it is mixed arterial and venous. I believe the arterial is used up in its passage through the placenta, so that when the blood reaches the interface with the maternal side, it has all been converted into venous, and all is then changed at the interface into arterial for the foetus and placenta. Diagrams 30 and 31.

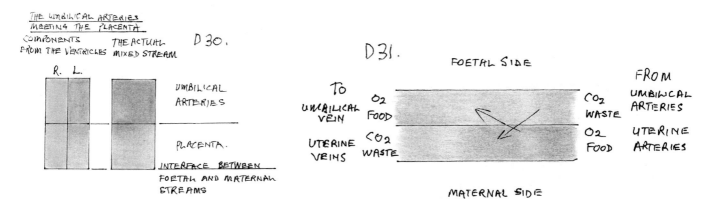

We can now see the whole plan of the circulation, with the upper and lower body sections and the placental section connected to the flyover and the junction. diagram 32.

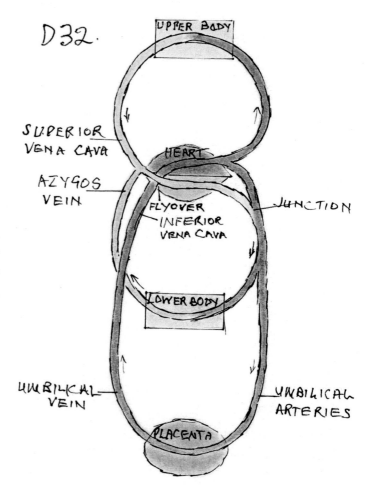

D32.

UPPER BODY

SUPERIOR VENA CAVA

AZYGOS VEIN

HEART

FLYOVER

INFERIOR VENA CAVA

JUNCTION

LOWER BODY

UMBILICAL VEIN

UMBILICAL ARTERIES

PLACENTA

The Foetal Lung.

Throughout the life of the foetus there are two respiratory organs in the circulation: the active placenta and the inactive foetal lungs. The blood supply for the placenta is large and the supply for the lungs small. With the latter, arterial is supplied by the bronchial arteries which arise from the upper aorta or its branches, while mixed venous and arterial is supplied by the pulmonary arteries which come off the pulmonary trunk, as I have shown earlier. The bronchial supply drains into the right atrium and the pulmonary into the left atrium. It is important for the lungs to be adequately supplied; they have to be in tip top condition and ready for the great day when they will play a vital key role instantly at the moment of birth. Diagram 33.

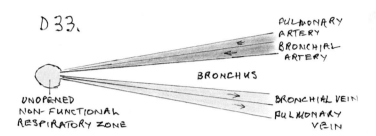

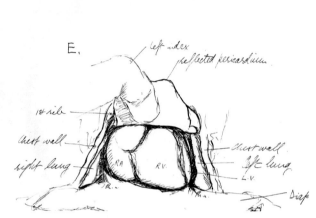

I have introduced another drawing, 'E', made in 1968 which shows the position of the unexpanded foetal lungs. Notice the phrenic nerves, Ph.n, and the tip of the left ventricle, LV peeping out from behind the right ventricle. Note also how the heart almost fills the whole chest. The finger is mine.

Summary of the foetal circulation.

The oxygen for the foetus comes from the placenta instead of the lungs, which are sidelined off the main circulation. There are three sections of the circulation, all connected to the heart: one for the upper body, one for the lower body and one for the placenta. The first has a rich supply of food and oxygen from the left side of the heart, while the other two receive a mixture of arterial from the left side and venous from the right. The mixed supply to the placenta is bigger than the supply to the lower body and carries most of the venous blood from the right heart to the placenta, where it is purified and returned to the left atrium of the foetal heart. The entrance to the left atrium is guarded by a valve, the foramen ovale, which ensures a constant flow of blood for the heart. The combined venous return from the upper and lower sections enters the right atrium and flows above the placental stream entering the left atrium in a 'flyover' manner. The streams of arterial and venous blood issuing from the ventricles meet at a junction to form the beginning of the descending aorta, which leads to the lower body and placenta. These two unique foetal features the flyover and the junction, form the foundation of the plan of the circulation and give it a beautiful simplicity, which allows it to change into that of the neonate within the space of one deep breath at the instant of birth.

Part 3. The Birth Changes.

A bright new light which illuminated the long hidden secrets of the foetus in April 1965, had been switched on by the death of the little girl who had failed to breathe after her delivery. Why she did not breathe we shall never know, but we will know that the transition from foetus to baby is due to the onset of breathing. The light is never switched on again, and we are kept in the dark during the transition. We can see the external changes: the waking, the breathing and the crying, but the internal changes are shielded from us and have never been seen. But if we have been able to recognise correctly how the foetus differs from the neonate, we will be more able to work out/guess the hidden changes which must occur at birth. As they depend on breathing they cannot occur in the mother; they take place outside the mother after the delivery. So the creature which is delivered is a foetus, and the birth of the baby takes place after the delivery on the delivery couch or in the midwife's arms as she is trying to clear the airway, when the first deep breath is taken. The little 'girl' who had died in 1965 would also have been a foetus, and it was her foetal features which had shone so brightly on that April day.

It is important to search for any clues which may help us to understand the internal changes which occur during the transition. But first of all we must consider the situation of the human foetus to be the same as that of the wild animal foetus, without the presence of any professional medical attendants to affect the outcome of the delivery (apart from the mother). So let us go to the beginning and start with the delivery. As it is completed the emptied contracted uterus will squash the placenta and stop the circulation within it and within all the vessels of the cord, and the foetus will be denied a blood supply. This is a clue: the first evidence of a possible change to the internal circulation of the foetus. There will be a double effect, with the stopping of the flow in the umbilical vein to the foetus, and the stopping of the flow in the umbilical arteries to the placenta. There may be a flow of oxygenated blood into the umbilical vein as the uterus mangles the placenta and wrings out the blood, and this may be of benefit for the foetus at this critical time if such a flow is able to reach the left atrium, but the loss of the placental circulation heralds the closure of the umbilical vein. The effect on the placenta will be more dramatic; there may be pulsation in the umbilical arteries but there can be no flow into the placenta. The large cardiac output of mixed blood for the placenta will be captured by the foetus and transferred to the lower body, returning as venous to the right atrium. So the foetus will gain from the effects on both the umbilical vein and the umbilical arteries, and will be well cared for naturally at this time before the delivery of the placenta.

Then the breathing begins. But when does it begin, and why does it begin? It is usually accompanied by the arrival of consciousness, we must not forget that. I believe there must be an inhibitory factor which prevents the foetus from waking and breathing in utero, and that after the delivery it is cancelled. Simultaneously another factor, stimulation, probably the shock of entry into the outside world, especially the rapid cooling of its wet naked body like having a cold shower, causes the foetus to wake and cry and breathe.

Here I must digress and expose some of my thoughts on respiration. I will not have another opportunity to talk about them, so I am taking the liberty of slipping them into this, my own little book. I have found it difficult to accept that the respiratory centre in the brain could analyse the level of carbon dioxide in the blood because its blood supply would have been purified already in its passage through the lungs, and it would be protected from the toxic effects of CO_2. So I presume there is a sensory centre *proximal* to the lungs which can detect the levels of CO_2 in the blood *before* it has passed through the lungs and relay information to the respiratory centre. In which case the system for respiratory control would consist of three parts: the outlying sensory centre proximal to the lungs, the control centre in the brain distal to the lungs receiving data from the sensory centre, and the lungs placed between the two. Now as I see it, and most of what I write is as I see it, the only sensible place in the circulation where the level of carbon dioxide could be measured satisfactorily would be in the right atrium, where there is a confluence of all the venous blood arriving from the peripheral tissues. But the sensory centre for the control of the cardiac output, the pacemaker, is also in the right atrium. So could the two be associated, or even be part of a single large sensory centre measuring both volume and quality of blood returning from the body? In which case the enlarged 'pacemaker' would control the heart rate and the respiratory rate, and any activity of the body causing an increased return of venous blood and carbon dioxide to the right atrium would be matched by a comparable increase of both the heart rate and the respiratory rate. The two would be synchronised and the control of the heart and respiratory rates would eventually be from the cardiac and respiratory centres in the brain stem.

Let us return to the foetus and continue to explore the birth changes.

Is it possible, I wonder, for the large amount of blood transferred from the blocked placenta to the right atrium, to be a factor in the initiation of respiration? Breathing may have started already before any appreciable change in the umbilical vessels, or may follow those changes. Either way I believe the following changes occur. They are all guess work of course, but I have had the benefit of seeing the two foundation stones which has helped me to work out the changes. They are difficult to describe in sequence because they occur simultaneously, and as we are dealing with circulatory changes they must inevitably involve pressure gradients, but they all depend on the expansion of the chest and the descent of the diaphragm, and all involve the left atrium. Especially important is the strong attachment of the inferior vena cava to the central tendon of the diaphragm; it is the place where circulatory and respiratory anatomy and physiology meet, and it ensures that the circulatory and respiratory changes at birth are perfectly synchronised.

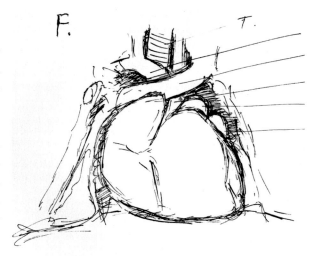

The chest has the shape of a cone with the diaphragm rising steeply from its sides to a highly placed central dome, and with the organs packed closely together above it contributing to the economy of space in the foetus. See my drawing 'F' of 22nd May 1968. When the first deep breath is taken the organs move down to a lower and wider section of the cone, which becomes even wider with the expansion of the chest wall, the diaphram becomes more flattened and there is a sudden increase in the size of the thoracic cage matched by a sudden decrease in the intra-thoracic pressure. Two fluid components allow the chest and lungs to expand: air entering the respiratory passages from the trachea, and venous blood entering the pulmonary arteries from the pulmonary trunk.

The inferior vena cava, strongly attached to the central tendon of the diaphragm, is pulled away from the atrial septum by the descending diaphragm and leads into the right atrium, while the left atrium loses its blood supply, and the foramen ovale closes, being exposed to both atria for the first time. The right atrium unrolls and acquires its second vena cava from the one discarded by the left atrium. (Now we see where the second vena cava comes from, and why it can now truly be called a vena cava). With the descent of the diaphragm, abdominal pressure is increased and thoracic pressure decreased, causing the lower venous return from the abdomen to enter the chest, while the pressure on the liver is removed, the blocked inferior vena cava opens and the venous return enters the right atrium and ventricle directly, with the return from the superior vena cava. The right ventricle responds to the increased volume of blood, and pumps the blood into the pulmonary trunk. The pressure in the trunk is high, possibly almost as high as that in the aorta, and there is a large pressure gradient between it and the lungs, which diverts the venous blood from the pulmonary trunk into the pulmonary arteries in the lungs.

This great diversion is a major event with a beneficial massive disruption of the circulation, giving the foetus a new life of independency from the mother, only comparable to life-threatening pathological events such as a pulmonary embolism. And it happens in the twinkling of an eye, invisibly in front of those who are privileged to witness the birth of a waking baby, when the first deep breath is taken. It suddenly removes the venous blood supply from three parts of the circulation: the ductus arteriosus, the lower body and the placenta, and directs it to the lungs. The ductus collapses without a blood supply and abolishes the segregated blood supply, and the umbilical arteries collapse too, while the lower body for a brief moment is left with a 50% reduced supply which is all arterial. If the first deep breath is taken before the transfer of blood from the placenta to the lower body, the major contribution of the blood diverted will come from the placenta with less from the lower body. But if there is any delay in the onset of breathing most diverted blood will come from the lower body with less from the placenta. Either way the total diverted will be away from the placenta and lower body. The diverted blood passes through the expanding lungs, becomes oxygenated and passes into the left atrium, left ventricle and aorta, and is distributed in full volume to both parts of the circulation at equalised pressure and speed. In the foetus the flow of mixed blood through the lungs would be small, but when the diverted blood arrives as the creature becomes a baby it would be a huge torrent of all the circulating blood.

It is great theatre: the left atrium occupies centre stage, with dissolution and assembly side by side in each wing.

On the right the descending diaphragm pulls the inferior vena cava away from the atrial septum, cutting off the arterial supply for the left atrium and closing the foramen ovale. The right atrium unrolls, obtains its second vena cava discarded by the left atrium and receives venous blood from both venae cavae which is pumped into the right ventricle and pulmonary trunk.

On the left there is the great diversion of the pulmonary trunk blood from the placenta and lower body to the expanding lungs, left atrium, left ventricle and aorta with an uninterrupted supply of oxygen for the changing creature, and the closure of the ductus arteriosus and distribution of arterial blood to both parts of the body at equalised pressure and speed.

The changeover from placental to pulmonary respiration and the changeover from placental to pulmonary blood in the left atrium have been safely accomplished. Diagram 34.

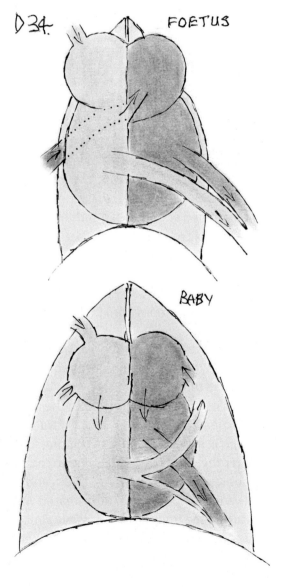

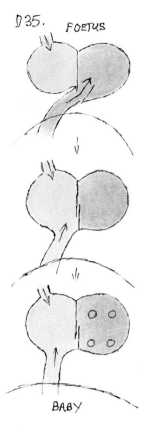

D35. FOETUS

BABY

In diagram 35, we can see several things: the descent and flattening of the diaphragm pulling the inferior vena cava away from the septum and stopping the blood supply to the left atrium, exposing the closing foramen ovale to the right atrium, which is acquiring its second vena cava discarded by the left atrium, now supplied by the four pulmonary veins.

Diagram 36, illustrates the great diversion from the placenta and lower body to the lungs with the first deep breath.

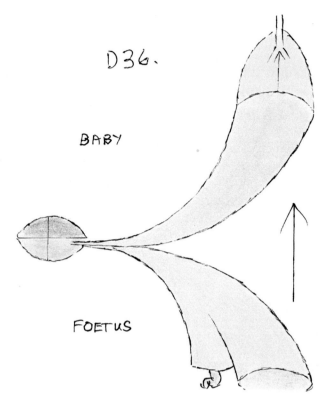

D36.

BABY

FOETUS

Diagram 37, shows the closing of the ductus arteriosus, the abolition of segregation between the upper and lower parts of the circulation, and the distribution of arterial blood to both parts.

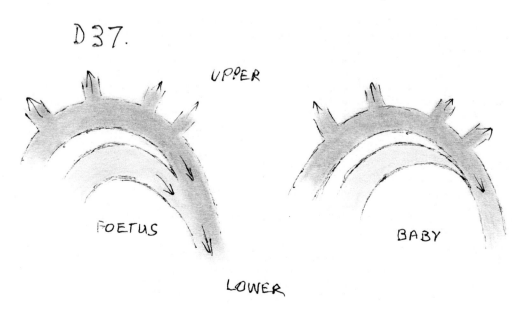

D37.

UPPER

FOETUS

LOWER

BABY

Diagram 38, shows the lung changes. With the baby I have shown the pulmonary arteries feeding the right lung, and the oxygenated blood returning from the left lung in the pulmonary veins to the left atrium. The collapsed and closed ductus is also shown.

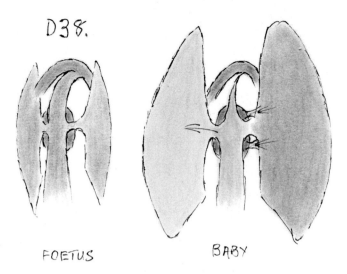

FOETUS   BABY

The connective and elastic tissue of the expanding lungs pull open the airways and pulmonary vessels, and blood flows side by side with air to the periphery where the exchanges of the respiratory gases occur.

In diagram 39 a, the outlines of the bronchi are shown. In b, the right pulmonary arteries are shown leading off the pulmonary trunk and carrying venous blood to the peripheral respiratory zone. The left lung has been divided into two parts. The outer part shows the pulmonary arteries reaching the respiratory zone with venous blood, and the inner part shows the pulmonary veins returning to the left atrium with oxygenated blood.

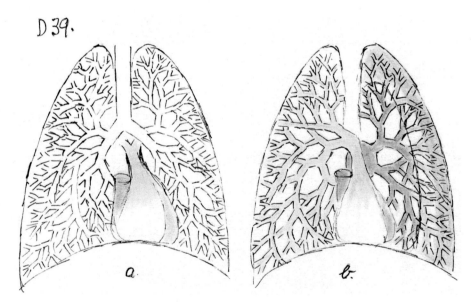

Diagram 40, shows the circulatory changes in the lower body during the transition from foetus to baby.

a). Foetus in utero.

b). Foetus after delivery, with transfer of blood in the descending aorta from placenta to lower body.

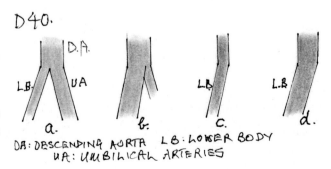

c). The creature in transition from foetus to baby with the first deep breath and loss of the venous portion during the great diversion

d). Baby after closure of the ductus arteriosus, with abolition of segregation and equalised flow of arterial blood to the upper and lower body.

Here I have introduced a composite diagram 41, showing four stages of the foetus and baby. With the dotted lines I have tried to show vessels and the left atrium within the heart. I did not want to clutter them up with numbers and letters from my shaky pen; so my explanations of them follow below.

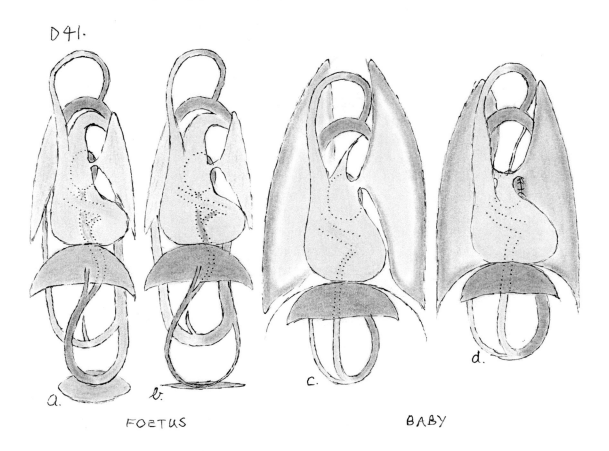

FOETUS   BABY

'a' represents the foetus in utero. It shows the umbilical vein leading to the liver and upper inferior vena cava, which is carrying the placental stream to the the left atrium and a small branch to the right atrium. The upper circulation contains mainly arterial blood from the left ventricle, while venous blood from the right ventricle is pumped up the pulmonary trunk to the ductus arteriosus to join the aortic flow. The mixed flow then passes down the descending aorta to the placenta and lower body. The lower venous return flows up the azygos vein to the right atrium while the mixed blood for the placenta is purified and enters the umbilical vein. The unexpanded lungs receive mixed mainly venous blood from the pulmonary trunk. The chest is narrow and the heart is horizontal above the raised diaphragm.

'b' shows the position after the delivery. The placenta has been squashed, with fresh blood passing up the umbilical vein, while the circulation for the placenta has been blocked and the blood diverted to the lower body and azygos vein.

'c' shows position at the end of the first deep inspiration, and the transition from foetus to baby. The chest has opened and the diaphragm has descended, filling the lungs with air and venous blood which have reached the peripheral respiratory zone, while inside the more vertical heart the unblocked vena cava has been pulled away from the left atrium and leads venous blood into the right atrium. This is the very moment when the right atrium gains its second vena cava. The great diversion has removed the venous blood supply; from the ductus arteriosus which has collapsed, from the placenta which has been delivered and removed, and from the lower body which receives a reduced flow of only arterial blood. The return from the lower body can now flow in both the inferior vena cava and azygos vein to the right atrium.

'd' marks the end of the first expiration with oxygenated blood returning from the periphery of the lungs to the left atrium. The chest is smaller and the diaphragm higher, with the heart less vertical than in 'c'. Both sections of the circulation are well supplied with arterial blood at equalised pressure and speed, while the ductus is represented by a rather elongated ligamentum arteriosum. Throughout the four stages the left atrium and upper body have been well supplied wth oxygen.

The closure of the foramen ovale is a trivial matter; the valve is now exposed to both atria beating on each side of it, and with little pressure difference between the two sides there will be little flow between them. In atrial systole the stronger left atrium will close the valve. Also, there would be a large pressure difference in atrial systole between the raised pressures in the atria and the low pressures in the dilating ventricles, which would encourage the blood flowing in the atria to pass directly into the ventricles rather than through the valve. Diagram 42.

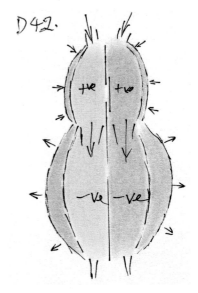

Various other reasons have been given for the closure of the ductus arteriosus. I would not disagree with some of them; it would seem that the ductus is primed ready for closure towards the end of the gestation period. But I believe the closure is eventually caused by the lack of a venous blood supply, with collapse of the empty sensitised vessel and closure by its strong elastic and muscle tissue.

I have indicated in previous paragraphs and diagrams that I consider the respiratory zone in the lung to be a peripheral one. I believe it to be so because movement of the lung is essential for respiration and most of the lung movement would be at the periphery. There would be no movement at the root of the lung, and between the root and the periphery there would be a gradient from no movement to much movement. Parallel with this gradient there would be another with from no respiratory tissues at the root to many at the periphery. If my description of the lung casts is a correct one, there would be more space between the bronchi and vessels in the lower lobes than in the upper lobes, which would allow more movement and better ventilation in the lower. Another observation was the veins not following the bronchi as closely as the arteries. The two are connected of course by the capillaries, so they must have a relationship not revealed after the destruction by acid of the intervening tissues, and in life the veins would be carrying oxygen away from the tissues around and between the bronchi.

There is another invisible change which involves the transfer of the cardiac output by the ventricles, from the foetus and placenta to the systemic and pulmonary circulations of the baby. One of the more impossible fantasies of some of the orthodox accounts has been the concept of right heart dominance in the foetus, where the right ventricle has more muscle than the left. It has even been alleged that after birth there is a gradual reshaping of the ventricles leading eventually to the normal larger left ventricle. There is no doubt that the normal foetal left heart has more muscle bulk than the right. It is confirmed in an important article by Calvin E. Oyer et al., from the departments of pathology and pediatrics, Women and Infants hospital, and Brown Medical School, Providence, Rhode Island, United States. Professor Oyer has kindly and freely alowed me to quote from it. It is a retrospective review of autopsy and surgical pathology reports of 776 fetuses and neonates during the period 1978 through2002. It states ' Mean left ventricular wall thickness is greater than mean right ventricular wall thickness throughout gestation.' During the last ten weeks of gestation the averages were 3.15mm for the right ventricles and 3.87mm for the left ventricles; a ratio of 1: 1.23 R: L. The same ratio would apply to the neonate, with a smooth transition at birth as the right ventricle feeds the lungs and the left ventricle pumps to the body. It also reflects the large amount of work the right ventricle must do to supply the lungs; almost as much as the left ventricle. To this must be added the work done by the left ventricle in supplying the respiratory muscles of the chest and diaphragm; perhaps 80% or more of the total cardiac output devoted to respiration at the time of birth. The adult ratio of the ventricular wall thicknesses is different: 1: 3 right to left ventricle, which indicates how the body will develop more than the respiratory system in the growth to adulthood.

The article from Professor Oyer not only condemns the concept of right heart dominance, but also shows the extra work the left heart must do compared with the work of the right heart. Here I am introducing a different plan of the circulation, with the two sides of the heart separated and with separation of the blood supply for the upper and lower parts of the foetus. I have also separated the mixed blood supply for the lower body and placenta into arterial and venous. Diagram 43. It shows clearly how only the lower body section is in parallel with that of the placenta; the upper circulation is without a parallel. In the previous version of my book I had worked out that the streams meeting at the junction were equal when considering the streams to be pure venous and pure arterial. But now that I know they are not pure, my reasoning loses some credibilty. However, it appears to me that the streams would be equal. In another version of my book I said ' The mixed blood flowing down the descending aorta must contain a sufficiently large arterial portion to support the life of the lower body. So I assume it would be at least 50% of the total.' Later I said 'If the mixed blood were more arterial than venous the lower limb would benefit but the placenta would be supplied with an unnecessarily high proportion of arterial, and not be able to purify enough venous. If the blood were more venous than arterial the lower limb would suffer and the placenta might not be able to cope with the large amount of venous. So I suppose a compromise has been reached where the balance is 50:50, or somewhere near that figure.'There are other things to consider. The venous return to the placenta represents the amount of oxygen used by the foetus. An equivalent amount of oxygen will be needed by the placenta to reverse this process and change the venous blood it receives into arterial, and the venous portion of the mixed stream must be matched by an equivalent portion of arterial to make this change. So I think we won't be far wrong if we consider them to be equal and it may help us to work out some of the haemodynamics. Diagram 43, is very helpful in this regard.

If we consider the circulation for the lower body, the venous portion has not come from the left ventricle; it has come from the right ventricle and passes through the lower body unchanged to the right atrium. It then circles round again indefinitely, adding to the venous return to the right heart which has come from the foetus supplied by the oxygenated blood from the left heart. So the total size of the right heart output equals the arterial supply to the foetus plus half the total supply to the lower body. We can now clearly see that the venous return to the placenta represents accurately the total arterial supply to the foetus, because the venous portion for the lower body has been excluded. If the streams at the junction are equal the arterial supply for the foetus, shown in red and represented by the venous return to the placenta, will equal the arterial supply for the placenta, and the total flow down the umbilical arteries will be double the arterial supply to the foetus. That is why the left heart has to do more work than the right heart; *because it has to supply the foetus and the placenta with equal amounts of arterial blood,* while the right heart pumps the venous return from the foetus plus the venous portion of the mixed supply to the lower body.

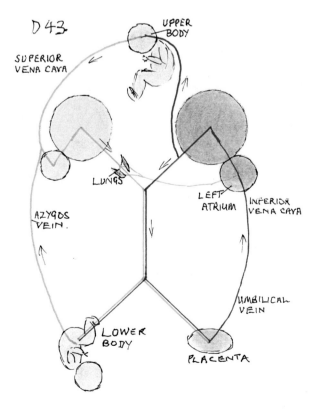

If the streams at the junction are equal the umbilical arteries will carry mixed blood into the placenta; half venous from the right heart which has come from the foetus to be purified, and half arterial from the left heart for the placenta itself. But not at the rate of 100%, only 50%, because only half of the total travels at twice the speed of the flows before the junction, as we can see from my traffic arrangement, where only 50% of the vehicles are able to travel after the junction at double the speed of the vehicles behind. The normal foetal heart rate is 140 beats per minute, twice that of the mother's heart. So the speed of the flows in the umbilical arteries would be extremely fast, double that of the flows before the junction, and the blood would pass from foetus to placenta in a very short time; which augurs well for the arteries as they have no source of oxygen and food apart from the blood rushing through them. Then the pace slackens and slows to the normal in the umbilical vein, where it is controlled by the beating of the left atrium and the foramen ovale at 140 beats per minute. This is still very fast, and it has to be, *because the left heart has to feed the foetus and the placenta with equal amounts of arterial blood*. It could do this either by pumping the total amount of blood with a double-sized heart at 70 beats per minute, or by pumping 50% of the blood at 140 beats with a normal heart. The latter option has been chosen; the heart cannot shrink suddenly at birth. Now we see why the foetal heart rate is so fast, and why it slows later after the placental circulation has been dismantled.

****

Delay in the onset of breathing.

There may be many reasons for delayed breathing, but in each case the result will be the same; each passing moment without breathing will threaten the life of the foetus, and urgent steps will need to be taken to avoid its death. I believe the foetus is able to endure an abnormally long period of apnoea because the only active part is the beating heart, but if spontaneous breathing does not occur active intervention will be needed. Three things will be required urgently: air in the lungs, blood in the lungs and movement in the lungs.

Bearing in mind my description of the circulation and the birth changes, let us try to imagine what might occur when there is delay in the onset of breathing after the delivery. The diaphragm of the foetus will be undescended, the foramen ovale will be covered by the upper inferior vena cava and the right atrium will be in the rolled up state. The great diversion from the pulmonary trunk to the lungs will not have occurred, no blood will have reached the left atrium from the unexpanded lungs, and when the supply from the umbilical vein will have stopped the left atrium will be denied a blood supply from each side; from the inferior vena cava and the lungs. The supply of oxygen and food for both sides of the heart from the coronary vessels will be reduced, the heart will weaken and the output from each ventricle will be reduced. If some blood is able to return to the right heart there may be some flow to the lower body of venous blood, but without a supply of arterial blood to the left heart the circulation on each side will weaken and slow. The slower heart will conserve energy, and with each deteriorating moment more slowing will mean more conservation until all reserves have been used up and the heart will stop beating.

Now the active management. The first thing to do, apart from clearing the airway of course, is to inflate the lungs, but it must be done as quickly and powerfully as with a normal birth to imitate the great diversion and flood the lungs with blood and air. As I see it, it could only be done properly by imitating the natural way by quickly and strongly reducing the pressure in the chest using a mini iron lung. It may not cause the foetus to start breathing, but it would put blood and air into the lungs, and artificial respiration would have to be carried out until the creature could breathe on its own. There may be other things to do, *but nothing would be more important than flooding the lungs with blood and air*. Puffing gently into the lungs might inflate them, but there would be positive pressure on the pulmonary vessels, not negative, without suction to fill them with blood;

though slowly and eventually the connective tissues of the lung would pull open the vessels with the same effect, after some time if death had not supervened.

Before I end this story I want to see why there has been such a difference between the orthodox accounts and my own; most importantly, why I have seen the placental stream leading to the foramen ovale and the left atrium, while others have seen it going to the right atrium. In 1968 when I was examining foetuses in the medical school, I had failed to find the uppermost part of the inferior vena cava attached to the atrial septum round the foramen ovale. So in each case the inferior cava led into the right atrium, as in the orthodox accounts. There may be several reasons for this. Perhaps the most likely being the sudden loss of muscle tone in the right atrial wall at death and the falling away from the septum by the inferior vena cava showing the postnatal position. Also, the foetus may have breathed just before death and changed the foetal arrangement into that of the neonate, with the inferior cava leading into the right atrium. In some cases the examining fingers may have disturbed the anatomy on opening the right atrium. Or perhaps it had just been assumed that the inferior vena cava led into the right atrium in the foetus as it does after birth. For whatever reason the inferior cava had not been found to enter the left atrium until April 1965 when I had seen it in the heart removed in the mortuary. I have recently confirmed this arrangement by examining the foetal lamb and showing you a picture of it.(No. 5). This was the uncovering of the most secret of the secrets of the hidden foetal circulation. Another uncovered secret was the absence of an inferior vena cava below the liver in the lamb. Those investigating the circulation with radiography could not have recognised this; they would have seen the blood streams, but the soft tissue details would have been radiolucent.

On 7th July 2018 I examined the heart, lungs and liver of a lamb, all connected and freshly acquired from the butcher in Oswestry. I confirmed there was no inferior vena cava below the liver. I exposed the inferior vena cava leading from the liver to the right atrium, and the superior vena cava leading to the right atrium from above. I opened the inferior vena cava and showed it leading to the pale scar of the closed foramen ovale known as the fossa ovalis. I then directed my incision to the left and opened the right atrium. Where there had been a small gap between the inferior vena cava and the right atrium in the foetal lamb, there was now a wide connection between that part which contained the fossa ovalis and the main part of the atrium, and the widened upper end of the inferior vena cava led to both. I opened the superior vena cava and showed it entering the right atrium from above. I took pictures at every stage.

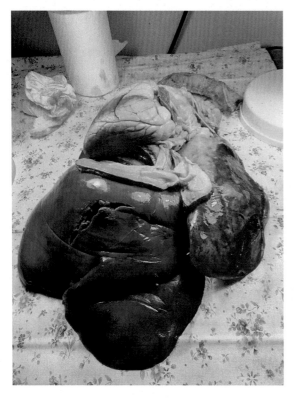

Picture 12

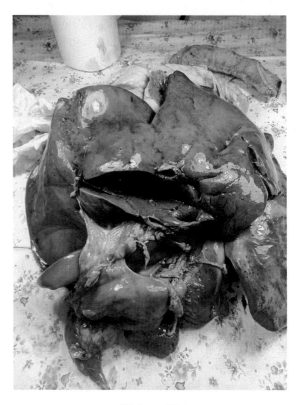

Picture 13

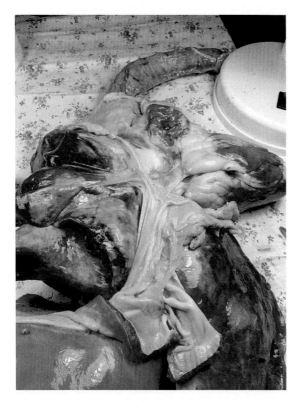

Picture 14

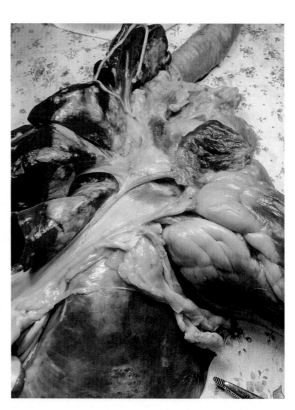

Picture 15

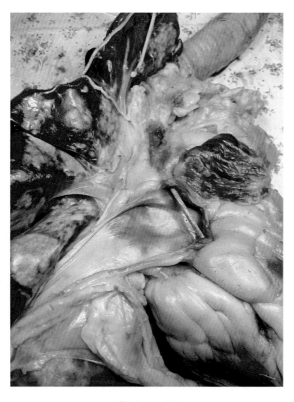

Picture 16

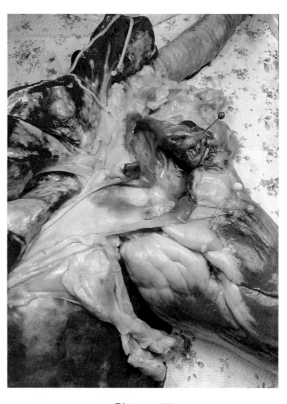

Picture 17

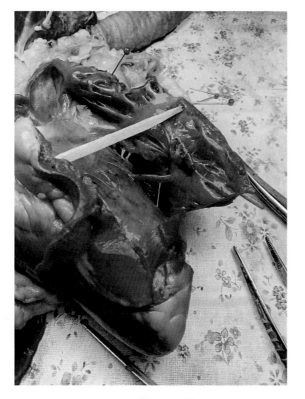

Picture 18

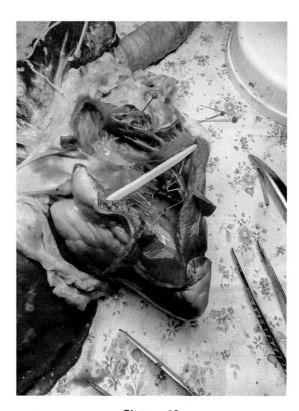

Picture 19

The pictures show: 12, the three organs, without a vena cava below the liver, and the vena cava above the liver leading to the heart. 13, Confirming the absence of a vena cava below the liver. 14, The vena cava above the liver leading from the liver and diaphragm to the right atrium. 15, The inferior vena cava opened showing part of the fossa ovalis, and leading into part of the right atrium.16, Part of the right atrium propped open with a stick showing the fossa ovalis. 17,The right atrium opened with the edges pinned back and both venae cavae opened and entering the atrium. 18 & 19, The opened right atrium and ventricle, with the dark recess at the side leading to the pulmonary trunk.

On considering these recent pictures of the lamb's anatomy and the one I had taken previously of the foetal lamb, I can now see why there has been such discord between us. The right atrium is really in two parts in both foetus and lamb. In the lamb we see both parts united with a large gap between the two and with the superior vena cava entering the larger part from above and the inferior vena cava leading into both parts from below. But in the foetus there is a partition between the two and the vena cava leads only into the smaller part with a small gap in the partition leading into the larger part. The inferior vena cava passes through the right atrium in a tunnel without entering the atrium except for the small part which branches off through the gap. It then leads to the foramen ovale at the end of the tunnel and leads the placental stream through the valve into the left atrium. So the placental stream leads to the right atrium and even passes through it in the inferior vena cava, *but does not enter it; the vena cava carries the stream right up to the foramen ovale and the stream passes through the valve into the left atrium.* Those investigating the foetal circulation with radiography would have been unable to see these important radiolucent details. In the human I have shown what I believe happens at birth, with the inferior vena cava pulled away from the septum and leading venous blood from the lower body into the right atrium. In the lamb it would seem that the main change would be the removal of the partition between both parts of the right atrium, with the inferior vena cava feeding an enlarged atrium with blood from the liver which had lost its placental contribution, while the superior vena cava would continue to supply the atrium with the total venous return. In the postnatal human the blood from the liver would mix with the venous blood in the inferior vena cava, but in the lamb the mixing would occur in the right atrium with the venous blood from the superior vena cava. In the lamb, as in the human, it would be the interatrial position of the foramen ovale at birth which would cause the valve to close. In the human I have assumed that it is the expansion of the chest and the descent of the diaphragm which cause the birth changes. Would they cause, or how would they cause the changes in the foetal lamb? Perhaps we should leave this problem and end the human story which has benefitted so much from exploring the lamb and foetal lamb.

Birds have a circulation similar to our own, (and similar wrong accounts of it), with a four chambered heart, a foramen ovale and a pair of lungs. The circulation in the chick embryo is also similar to that of the human foetus, with the allantois, a membrane lining the inside of the egg shell, constituting the respiratory organ. I would suggest therefore that the foetal circulation could be investigated using fertilised hens' eggs. Bit by bit, piece by piece, slice by slice the mysteries of the circulation in the chick and foetus could be unravelled. Even more exciting; we will be able to uncover all those changes at birth that I have only been able to guess at. They will be revealed to us; the changes, not only in the chick but in ourselves. The work is waiting to be done. I am unable to do it, but someone will do it someday.

****

Picture 20, is of my father when he was younger. My mother's picture, 22, is opposite. In the centre in picture 21, taken in 1964 a year after our marriage, is my wife Pauline.

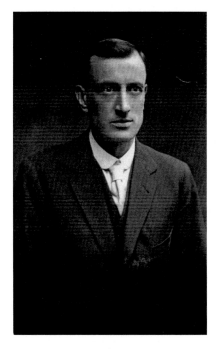 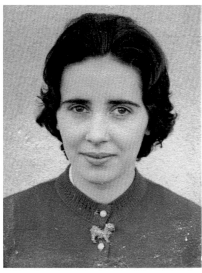 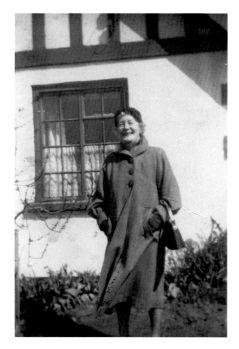

Picture 20   Picture 21   Picture 22

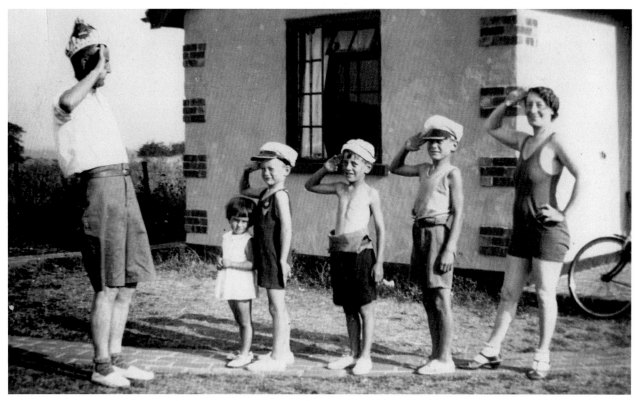

Picture, 23, is of my parents and the family taken during a summer holiday in 1932 or '33.

From left; Dad, Janet, Neil, Alan, Jim and Mum. We had been to the
Whitstable Carnival the day before, hence the hats.

Printed in the United States
By Bookmasters